Log Book

Aesth
TAPING
on face

MW00907175

This book belongs to: _____

Course by: _____   Date: _____

Kinesiology Tape I've tried	IImpressions	Notes

Where does the kinesiology taping method come from?

Kinesiology taping is a neuromuscular therapeutic method invented in the late 1970s by Dr. Kenzo Kase, a Japanese chiropractor, in response to limitations with rigid sports taping for his patients.

Thanks to its effectiveness, Dr. Kase's method has spread over the years all over the world, mainly in physiotherapy with important results for all types of patients and ages.

This method has revolutionized the world of rehabilitation and sports medicine. The correct application of the tape allows a considerable optimization and improvement of rehabilitation treatments and pain relief.

The basis of the taping method is the principle of "decompression" which facilitates improved movement and resolution of edema (the accumulation of fluid within the tissues).

What is beauty taping

Given the therapeutic effectiveness of the kinesiology taping method on the body, in recent years specific techniques have been developed for the aesthetic treatment of the face and neck that have shown excellent results with clear effects such as lifting, relaxing, smoothing, filling, detoxifying, draining and decontracting.

The application of kinesiology tape is extremely valid when used alone or in combination with other techniques to enhance its effects, such as in combination with manual massage therapy, facial gymnastics, aesthetic cupping, application of cosmetic products, cross taping, and so on.

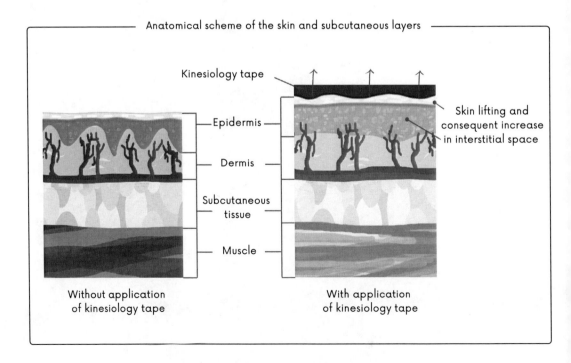

Anatomical scheme of the skin and subcutaneous layers

Kinesiology tape

Epidermis

Skin lifting and consequent increase in interstitial space

Dermis

Subcutaneous tissue

Muscle

Without application of kinesiology tape

With application of kinesiology tape

What is the kinesiology tape and how it works on the face

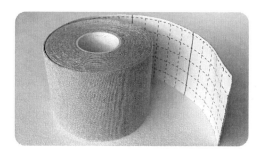

The kinesiology tape is an elastic cotton bandage with a medical hypoallergenic adhesive base that ensures skin breath-ability without leaving residue.

It contains no active ingredients inside. Its effectiveness is due to the special technology that uses a coefficient of elasticity, which imitates that of the skin, and a medical glue that allows a specific adherence to the skin; This produces a bio-mechanical decompression action that affects the haemo-lymphatic and muscular systems.

The part covered by the kinesiology tape lifts the skin, increasing the interstitial space: the pressure decreases, the lymphatic and blood circulation flows more easily, bringing more oxygen into the connective tissues and eliminating toxins. As a result, the cellular metabolism and the healing process of the tissues increases promoting the regeneration of elastic fibers and hyaluronic acid. Beauty kinesiology taping also has an important de-contracting effect on the mimic muscles in hypertonus, which cause the appearance of wrinkles and sagging skin.

With constant and specific applications, this technique obtains long-term results because they work on the correction and re-education of the muscles (the muscle regains its natural state of elongation and restores the correct volumes of the face, reducing wrinkles and redefining the contours).

Main effects of beauty taping

- Instant lifting effect.
- Redefinition of facial contours.
- Double chin reduction.
- Muscle re-education.
- Re-education of facial expressions.
- Age and expression wrinkles smoothed out.
- Hemolymphatic drainage
- Detoxification.
- Microcirculation stimulation.
- Skin more hydrated toned and elastic.
- Less visible scars.

What is cross taping and how does it work

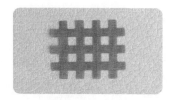

Cross taping is an inelastic, hypoallergenic, adhesive polyester patch in the shape of a quadrangular grid invented by a Korean physiatrist, Dr. Aeo Kang, and a Japanese osteopath, Nobutaka Tanaka.

The principle of cross taping is based on the concepts of traditional Chinese medicine. Its function is to generate a neuromuscular stimulation able to re-balance and stabilize the energy flow.

Cross taping therapy can be performed alone or in combination with kinesiology taping. Cross taping can be applied at strategic points of structural tension to reduce muscle spasm at the connection with the bone.

Prolonged spasmodic contractions of the facial expression muscles (facial spasm) can be caused by emotional stimuli, anxiety, stress, expression habits, and so on. The spasmodic and prolonged contraction of the mimic muscles is one of the main causes that over time causes the appearance of signs of aging such as wrinkles, loss of tone, change in facial volumes, and so on.

Manual massage techniques and specific applications of cross taping and kinesiology taping help muscle re-education and relaxation with consequent improved aesthetic effects on the face and neck.

As in kinesiology taping, the application of cross taping lifts the skin by decreasing interstitial pressure, relieving pain and helping drainage and decompression; in this way, positive effects are produced on muscle tone, hemo-lymphatic drainage and micro-circulation.

The application of cross taping is also indicated to re-establish the bioelectric balance and the micro electromagnetic currents that cross the skin, improving the functioning in cases of imbalance both at superficial and deep level.

Main Effects of cross taping applications:

Analgesic, muscle tone, hemo-lymphatic drainage and micro-circulation, Neuro reflex effects.

Cross taping is applicable upon:

- Painful area
- Acupuncture Points
- Trigger points
- Tender points
- Meridians

General side effects

When applied on healthy skin, kinesiology taping and cross taping are generally free of side effects. If in doubt, consult your doctor or therapist before application.

Never apply kinesiology tape or cross taping in the presence of:

- High fever
- Skin injuries
- Open or bleeding wounds
- State of immunodeficiency
- Tumors
- Ongoing allergic states
- Dermatitis

Tips for kinesiology taping

- Use a high-quality, facial-specific kinesiology tape that is latex-free and made of hypoallergenic materials.
- Use the kinesiology tape in the roll format of 5 meters by 5 cm to be cut to size according to the application to be made.
- Never apply kinesiology tape to injuries or irritated skin.
- Kinesiology tape can be applied day or night.
- Use very sharp scissors to cut kinesiology tape.
- Test the kinesiology tape on a small area beforehand to check for any allergic reactions.
- Stop applying kinesiology tape immediately if skin irritation or allergies occur.
- Kinesiology tapes can be used on the body up to 7 days, but on the face is recommended a maximum time of 24 hours and a minimum of 30 minutes. This time varies depending on the application you want to perform and your skin type.

General indications for kinesiology taping applications

- Perform the applications strictly following the instructions of your therapist or technician specializing in aesthetic kinesiology taping to avoid unwanted effects.
- A mild skin reaction is considered normal if it disappears within 30 minutes of tape removal, leaving no irritation or other kind of abnormal marks on the skin. If in doubt, consult your doctor or therapist.
- Clean and dry skin thoroughly before application.
- Apply the tape lengthwise following the elasticity of the fabric.
- Apply the tape with zero tension; stretching may create a compressive effect and generate the opposite effect as well as folds in the skin.

- Always attach the anchor without stretching or adding tension to the tape and muscle tissues.
- In the case of lifting applications, once the anchor is in place, stretch the muscles and then attach the rest of the tape without adding tension.
- In the case of lymphatic drainage applications, apply both the anchor and the rest of the tape without bringing the muscles and tape into stretch or tension.
- The tape should be removed gently by holding the tissues to one side and pulling the tape parallel to the skin at a 180° angle in the direction of the anchor. To facilitate removal the tape can be wet with tepid water.
- The tape is single-use.
- It is recommended not to exceed three applications at one time.

How to proceed - General information

1. Measure the tape before cutting it according to the area to be treated and according to your anatomy.

2. Cut the tape according to the directions of the application to be made, and round off the corners.

3. Peel off the tape paper at the point of the anchor for about 1 or 2 cm.

4. Attach the anchor to the face without stretching the tape or muscle tissue.

5. Peel off the rest of the paper keeping only a small portion at the end so that your fingers do not touch the adhesive part.

6. Place tape on skin according to application directions.

7. Once applied, rub the tape with your hands lengthwise in the direction of the anchor to attach it to the tissues and activate it.

8. Leave on according to the time indicated by your application.

9. To remove it, lightly hold the fabrics and pull it off at a 180 degree angle in the direction of the anchor. To facilitate the removal, you can wet the tape with warm water before removing it.

Head and neck muscles

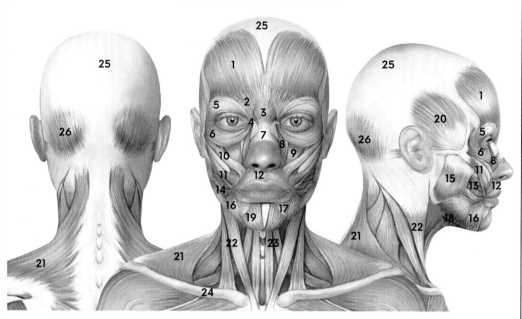

1. Frontalis
2. Corrugator supercilii
3. Procerus
4. Depressor supercilii
5. Orbicularis oculi superior
6. Orbicularis oculi lateral
7. Nasalis
8. Levator labii superioris alaeque nasi
9. Levator labii superioris
10. Zygomaticus minor
11. Zygomaticus major
12. Orbicularis oris
13. Buccinator
14. Risorius
15. Masseter
16. Depressor anguli oris
17. Depressor labii inferioris
18. Platysma
19. Mentalis
20. Temporalis
21. Trapezius
22. Sternocleidomastoid
23. Sternohyoid
24. Clavicle
25. Galea aponeurotica
26. Occipital

Table 1

Face and neck muscles - Main signs of expression and ageing

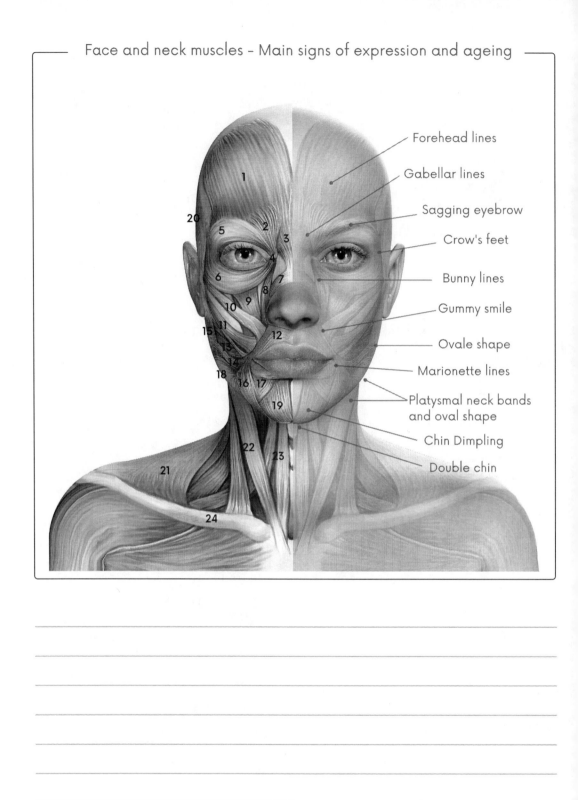

Forehead lines

Gabellar lines

Sagging eyebrow

Crow's feet

Bunny lines

Gummy smile

Ovale shape

Marionette lines

Platysmal neck bands and oval shape

Chin Dimpling

Double chin

Table 2

Lymph nodes scheme

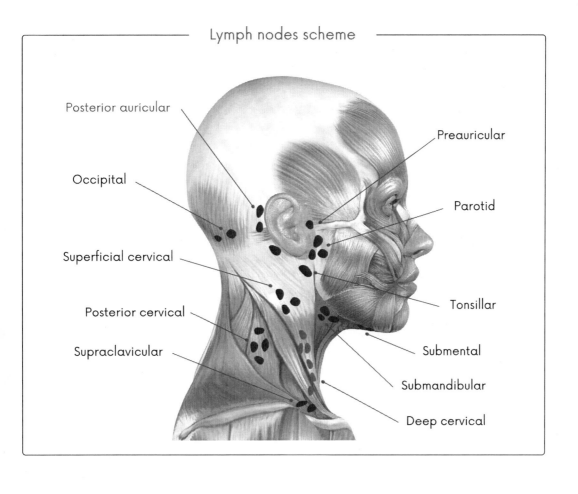

Posterior auricular

Occipital

Superficial cervical

Posterior cervical

Supraclavicular

Preauricular

Parotid

Tonsillar

Submental

Submandibular

Deep cervical

Table 3

Skull scheme

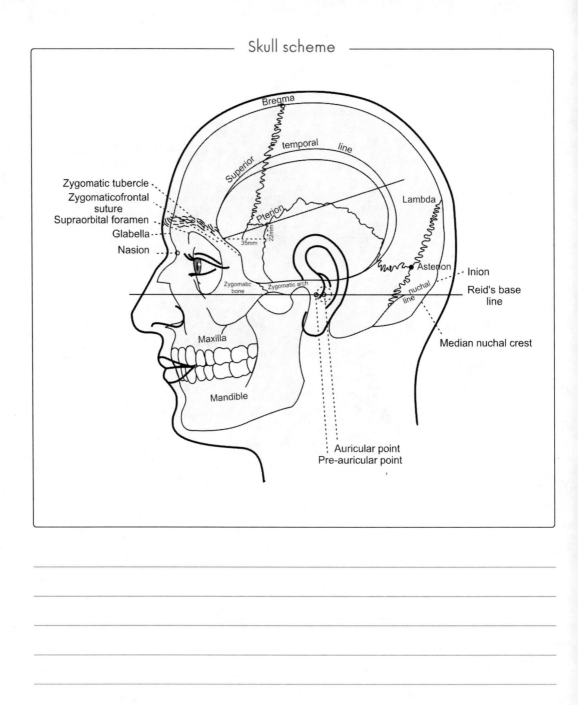

Bregma

temporal line

Superior

Lambda

Zygomatic tubercle
Zygomaticofrontal suture
Supraorbital foramen
Glabella
Nasion

Pterion

35mm

22mm

Asterion — Inion

Zygomatic bone

Zygomatic arch

nuchal line

Reid's base line

Maxilla

Median nuchal crest

Mandible

Auricular point
Pre-auricular point

Table 4

Skull anatomy

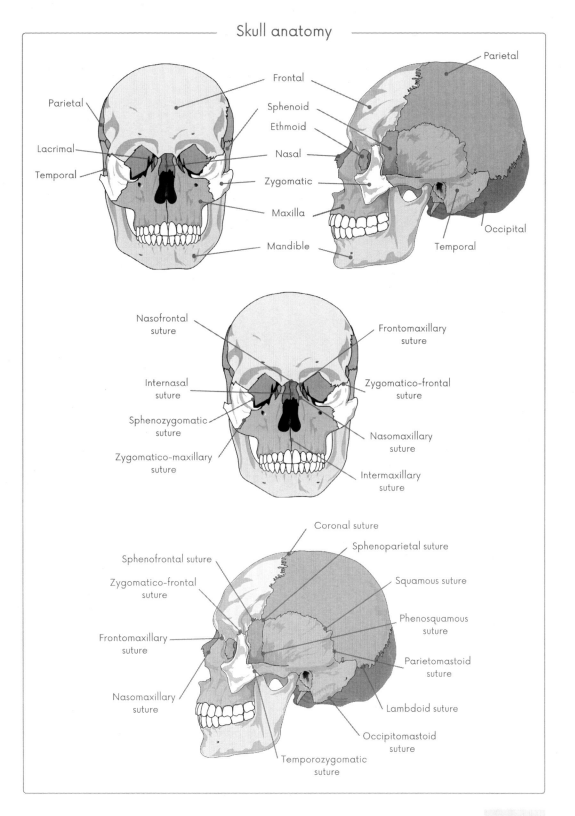

Table 5

Notes

Mark the muscles involved

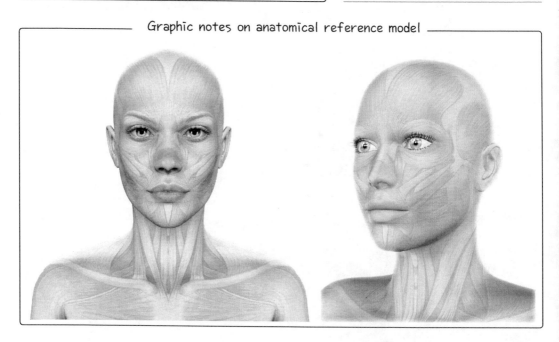

Muscles involved: _____

_____

_____

Application for: _____

_____

_____

_____

Effect: _____

_____

Graphic notes on anatomical reference model

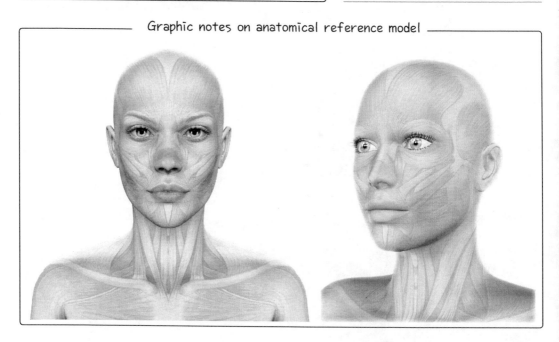

Photo

Graphic notes

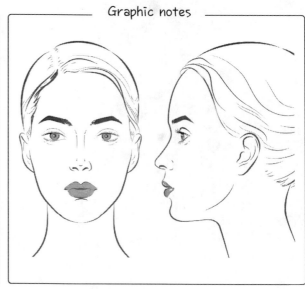

Tape: Quantity _____ Length _____ Width _____ N°Fingers _____ Width. Fingers _____

───────────── Draw the tape ─────────────

How to apply it: _____

_____

_____

_____

_____

_____

_____

_____

_____

_____

_____

_____

_____

_____

Notes: _____

_____

_____

_____

Mark the muscles involved

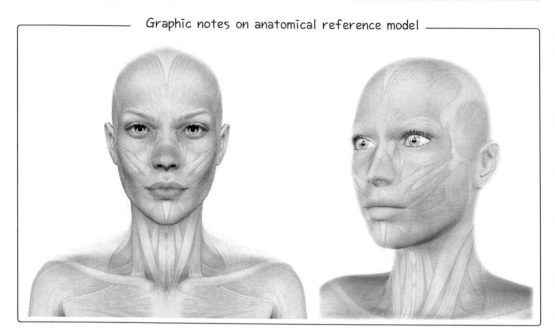

Muscles involved: _____
_____
_____

Application for: _____
_____
_____
_____

Effect: _____
_____

Graphic notes on anatomical reference model

Photo

Graphic notes

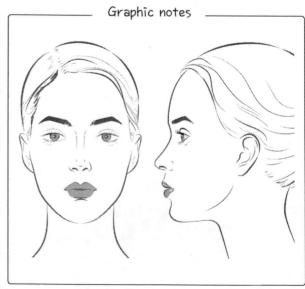

Tape: Quantity _____ Length _____ Width _____ N°Fingers _____ Width. Fingers _____

———————— Draw the tape ————————

How to apply it: _____

_____

_____

_____

_____

_____

_____

_____

_____

_____

_____

_____

_____

_____

_____

_____

Notes: _____

_____

_____

_____

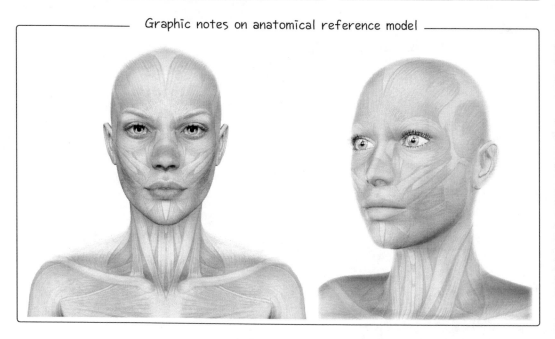

Muscles involved: _____
_____
_____
_____

Application for: _____
_____
_____
_____

Effect:_____
_____

Graphic notes on anatomical reference model

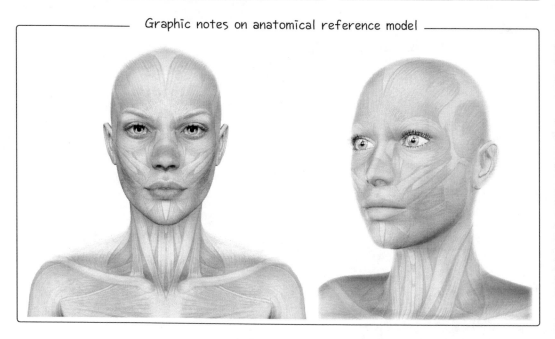

Photo

Graphic notes

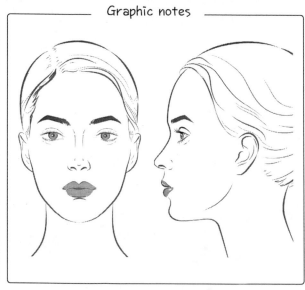

Tape: Quantity _____ Length _____ Width _____ N°Fingers _____ Width. Fingers _____

——————————————— Draw the tape ———————————————

How to apply it: _____

_____

_____

_____

_____

_____

_____

_____

_____

_____

_____

_____

_____

_____

_____

Notes: _____

_____

_____

_____

Mark the muscles involved

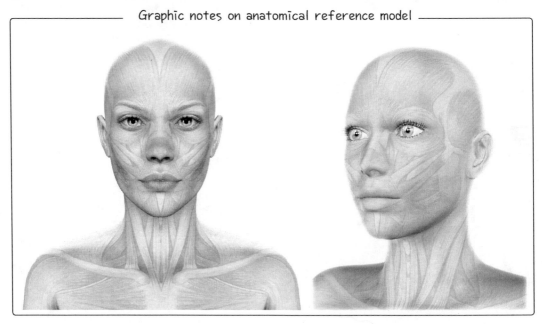

Muscles involved: _____

_____

_____

Application for: _____

_____

_____

_____

Effect:_____

_____

Graphic notes on anatomical reference model

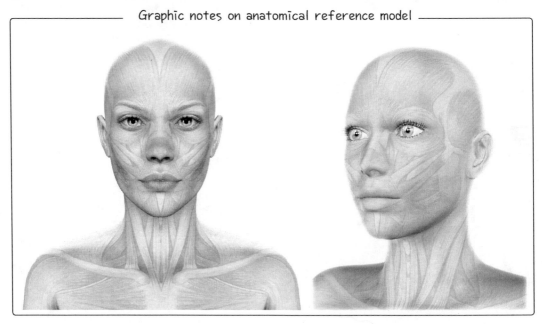

Photo

Graphic notes

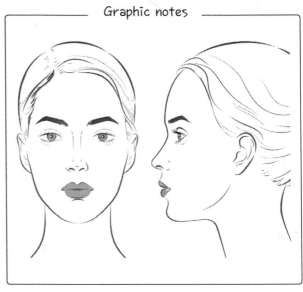

Tape: Quantity _____ Length _____ Width _____ N°Fingers _____ Width. Fingers _____

─────── Draw the tape ───────

How to apply it: _____

_____

_____

_____

_____

_____

_____

_____

_____

_____

_____

_____

_____

_____

_____

_____

Notes: _____

_____

_____

_____

Mark the muscles involved

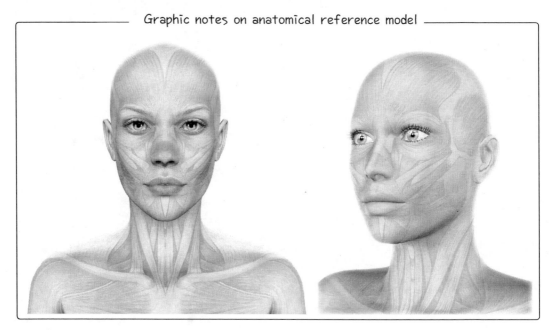

Muscles involved: _____

_____

_____

Application for: _____

_____

_____

_____

Effect: _____

_____

Graphic notes on anatomical reference model

Photo

Graphic notes

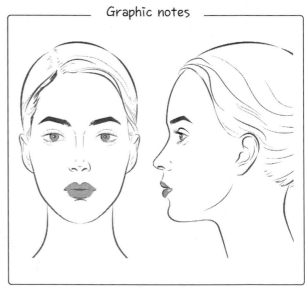

Tape: Quantity _____ Length _____ Width _____ N°Fingers _____ Width. Fingers _____

_____ Draw the tape _____

How to apply it: _____

_____

_____

_____

_____

_____

_____

_____

_____

_____

_____

_____

_____

_____

Notes: _____

_____

_____

_____

Mark the muscles involved

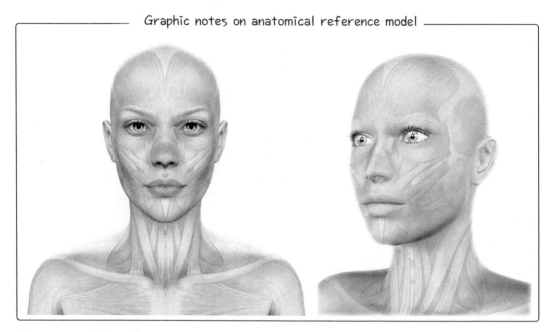

Muscles involved: _____
_____
_____

Application for: _____
_____
_____
_____

Effect: _____
_____

Graphic notes on anatomical reference model

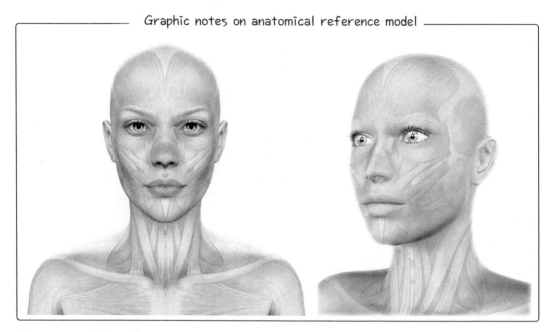

Photo

Graphic notes

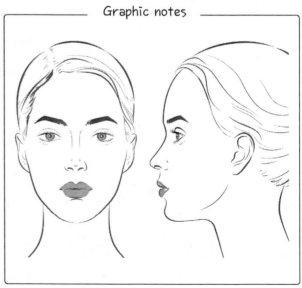

Tape: Quantity _____ Length _____ Width _____ N°Fingers _____ Width. Fingers _____

───────────────── Draw the tape ─────────────────

How to apply it: _____

_____

_____

_____

_____

_____

_____

_____

_____

_____

_____

_____

_____

_____

Notes: _____

_____

_____

_____

Mark the muscles involved

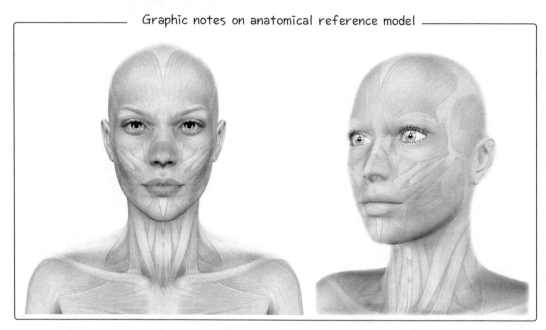

Muscles involved: _____

_____

_____

Application for: _____

_____

_____

_____

Effect: _____

_____

Graphic notes on anatomical reference model

Photo

Graphic notes

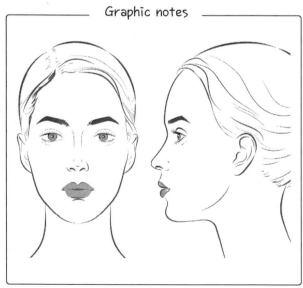

Tape: Quantity _____ Length _____ Width _____ N°Fingers _____ Width. Fingers _____

─── Draw the tape ───

How to apply it: _____

_____

_____

_____

_____

_____

_____

_____

_____

_____

_____

_____

_____

_____

Notes: _____

_____

_____

_____

Mark the muscles involved

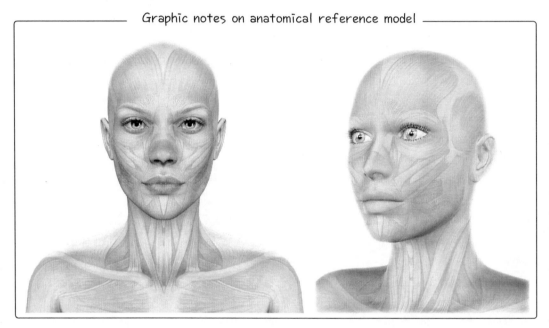

Muscles involved: _____

_____

_____

Application for: _____

_____

_____

_____

Effect:_____

_____

Graphic notes on anatomical reference model

Photo

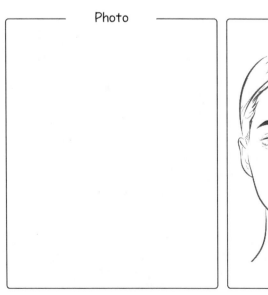

Graphic notes

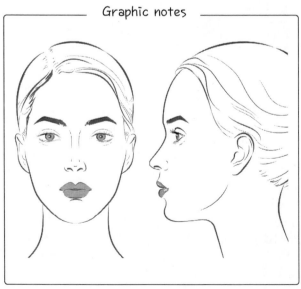

Tape: Quantity _____ Length _____ Width _____ N°Fingers _____ Width. Fingers _____

--- Draw the tape ---

How to apply it: _____

_____
_____
_____
_____
_____
_____
_____
_____
_____
_____
_____
_____
_____
_____
_____

Notes: _____

_____
_____
_____

Mark the muscles involved

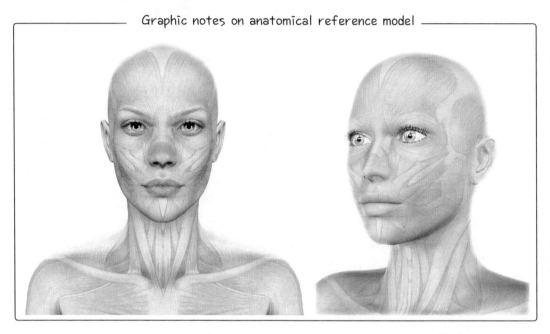

Muscles involved: _____

_____

_____

Application for: _____

_____

_____

_____

Effect: _____

_____

Graphic notes on anatomical reference model

Photo

Graphic notes

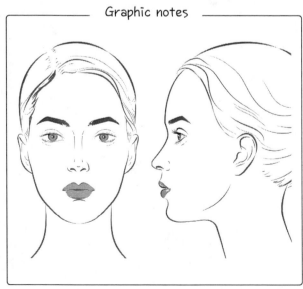

Tape: Quantity _____ Length _____ Width _____ N°Fingers _____ Width. Fingers _____

—— Draw the tape ——

How to apply it: _____

_____

_____

_____

_____

_____

_____

_____

_____

_____

_____

_____

_____

_____

Notes: _____

_____

_____

_____

Mark the muscles involved

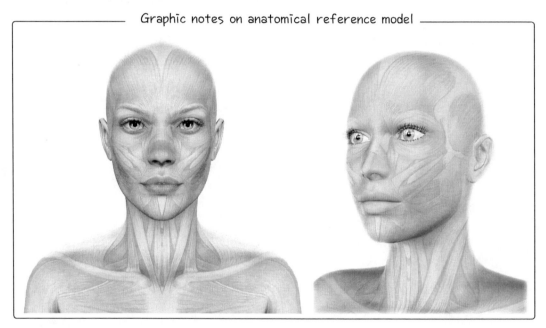

Muscles involved: _____
_____
_____

Application for: _____
_____
_____
_____

Effect: _____
_____

Graphic notes on anatomical reference model

Photo

Graphic notes

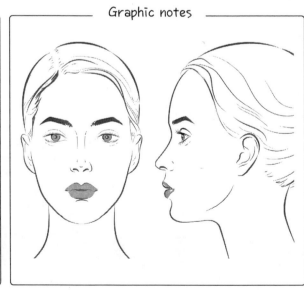

Tape: Quantity _____ Length _____ Width _____ N°Fingers _____ Width. Fingers _____

─────────── Draw the tape ───────────

How to apply it: _____

_____

_____

_____

_____

_____

_____

_____

_____

_____

_____

_____

_____

_____

Notes: _____

_____

_____

_____

Mark the muscles involved

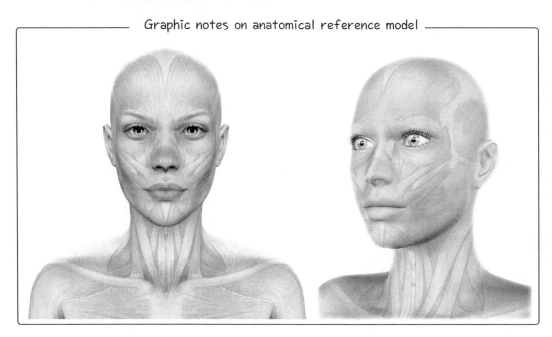

Muscles involved: _____
_____
_____

Application for: _____
_____
_____
_____

Effect:_____
_____

Graphic notes on anatomical reference model

Photo

Graphic notes

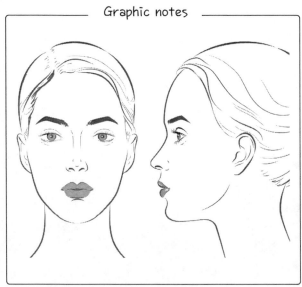

Tape: Quantity _____ Length _____ Width _____ N°Fingers _____ Width. Fingers _____

─────────────── Draw the tape ───────────────

How to apply it: _____

_____

_____

_____

_____

_____

_____

_____

_____

_____

_____

_____

_____

_____

Notes: _____

_____

_____

_____

Mark the muscles involved

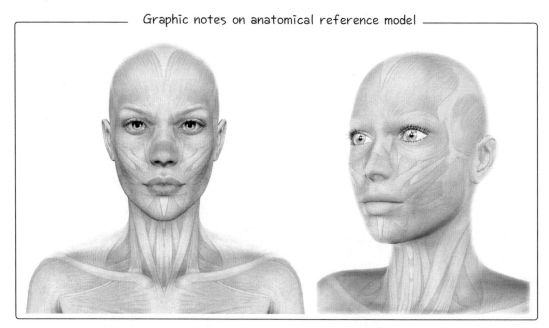

Muscles involved: _____
_____
_____

Application for: _____
_____
_____
_____

Effect: _____
_____

Graphic notes on anatomical reference model

Photo

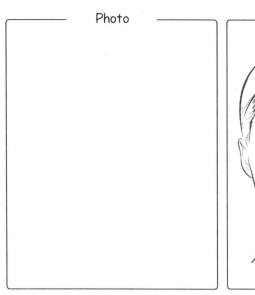

Graphic notes

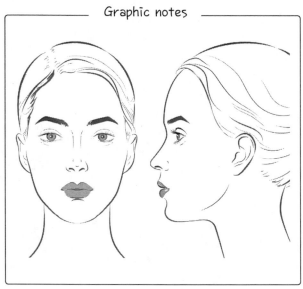

Tape: Quantity _____ Length _____ Width _____ N°Fingers _____ Width. Fingers _____

─────────────────── Draw the tape ───────────────────

How to apply it: _____

_____

_____

_____

_____

_____

_____

_____

_____

_____

_____

_____

_____

_____

Notes: _____

_____

_____

_____

Mark the muscles involved

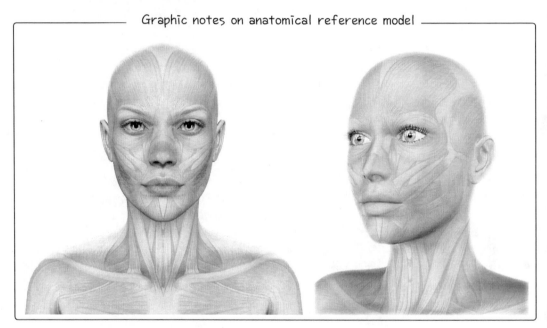

Muscles involved: _____

_____

_____

Application for: _____

_____

_____

_____

Effect:_____

_____

Graphic notes on anatomical reference model

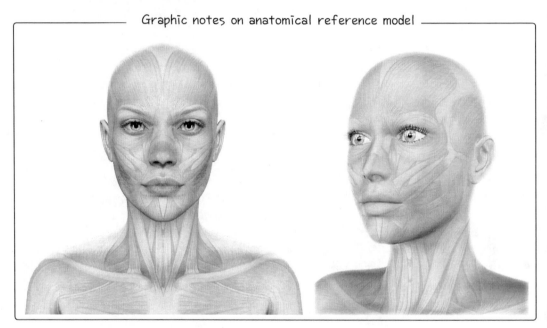

Photo

Graphic notes

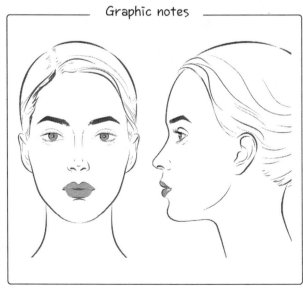

Tape: Quantity _____ Length _____ Width _____ N°Fingers _____ Width. Fingers _____

─────────────── Draw the tape ───────────────

How to apply it: _____

_____

_____

_____

_____

_____

_____

_____

_____

_____

_____

_____

_____

Notes: _____

_____

_____

_____

Mark the muscles involved

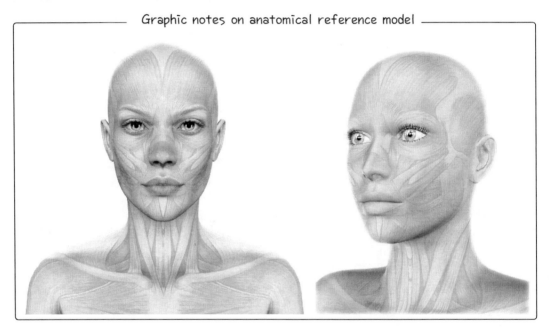

Muscles involved: _____

_____

_____

Application for: _____

_____

_____

_____

Effect:_____

_____

Graphic notes on anatomical reference model

Photo

Graphic notes

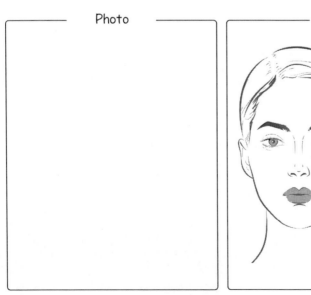

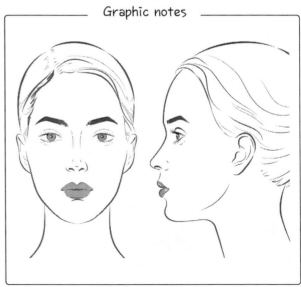

Tape: Quantity _____ Length _____ Width _____ N°Fingers _____ Width. Fingers _____

──────────────── Draw the tape ────────────────

How to apply it: _____

_____
_____
_____
_____
_____
_____
_____
_____
_____
_____
_____
_____
_____
_____
_____

Notes: _____
_____
_____
_____

Mark the muscles involved

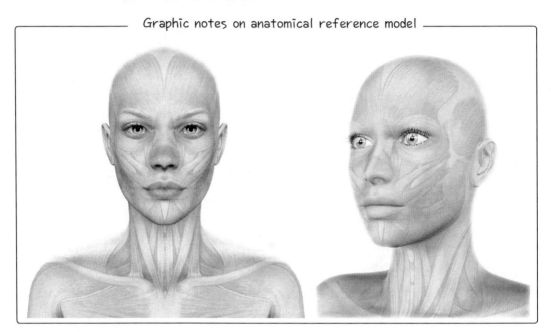

Muscles involved: _____
_____
_____

Application for: _____
_____
_____
_____

Effect: _____
_____

Graphic notes on anatomical reference model

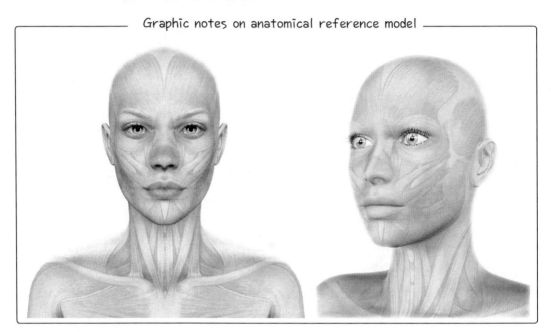

Photo

Graphic notes

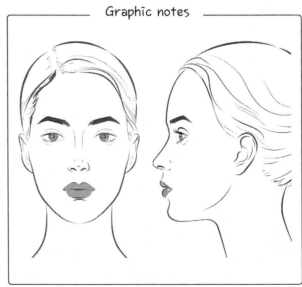

Tape: Quantity _____ Length _____ Width _____ N°Fingers _____ Width. Fingers _____

──────────── Draw the tape ────────────

How to apply it: _____

_____

_____

_____

_____

_____

_____

_____

_____

_____

_____

_____

_____

_____

_____

Notes: _____

_____

_____

_____

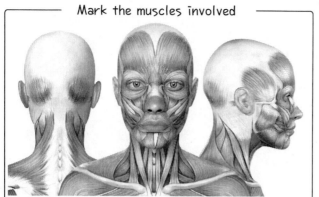

Muscles involved: _____
_____
_____

Application for: _____
_____
_____
_____

Effect: _____
_____

Graphic notes on anatomical reference model

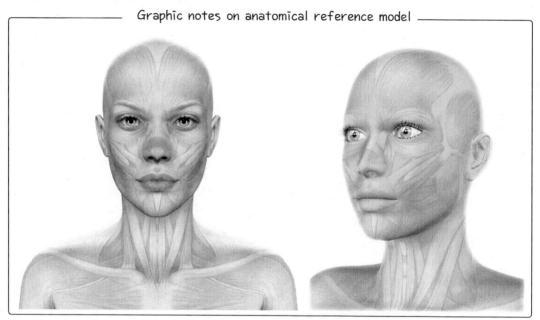

Photo

Graphic notes

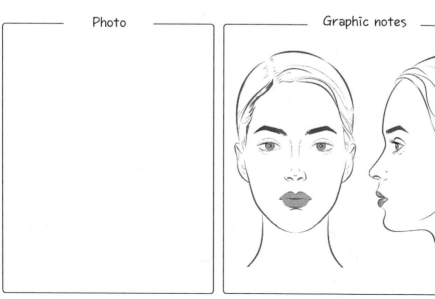

Tape: Quantity _____ Length _____ Width _____ N°Fingers _____ Width. Fingers _____

――――――――――― Draw the tape ―――――――――――

How to apply it: _____

_____

_____

_____

_____

_____

_____

_____

_____

_____

_____

_____

_____

_____

_____

Notes: _____

_____

_____

_____

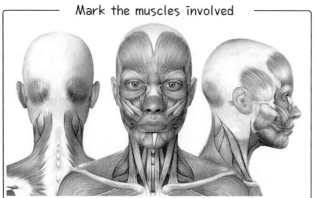

Muscles involved: _____
_____
_____

Application for: _____
_____
_____
_____

Effect: _____
_____

Graphic notes on anatomical reference model

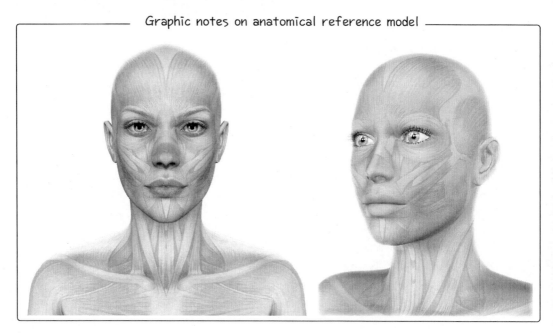

Photo

Graphic notes

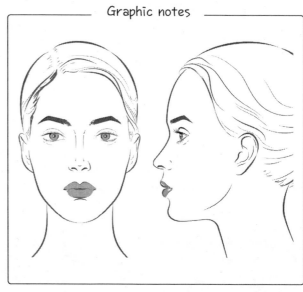

Tape: Quantity _____ Length _____ Width _____ N°Fingers _____ Width. Fingers _____

─────────── Draw the tape ───────────

How to apply it: _____

_____

_____

_____

_____

_____

_____

_____

_____

_____

_____

_____

_____

_____

Notes: _____

_____

_____

_____

Mark the muscles involved

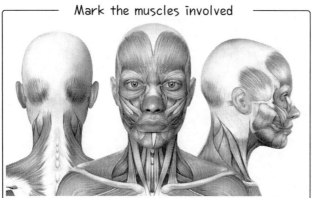

Muscles involved: _____
_____
_____

Application for: _____
_____
_____
_____

Effect: _____
_____

Graphic notes on anatomical reference model

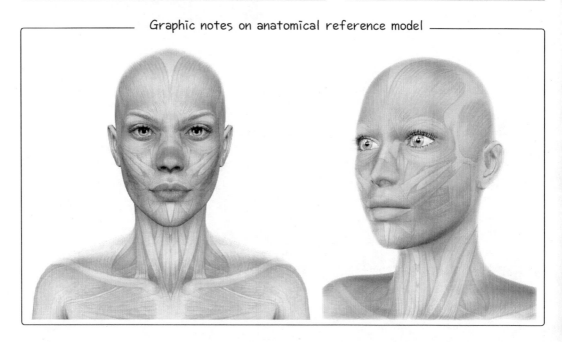

Photo

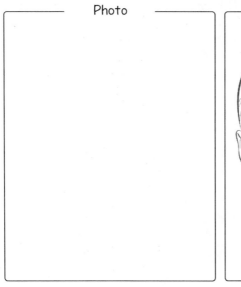

Graphic notes

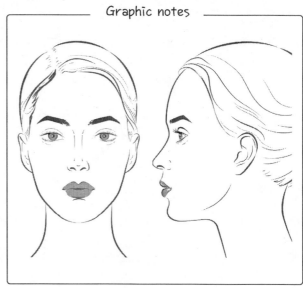

Tape: Quantity _____ Length _____ Width _____ N°Fingers _____ Width. Fingers _____

---------------------------------- Draw the tape ----------------------------------

How to apply it: _____

_____

_____

_____

_____

_____

_____

_____

_____

_____

_____

_____

Notes: _____

_____

_____

_____

Mark the muscles involved

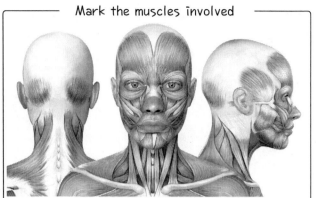

Muscles involved: _____

_____

_____

Application for: _____

_____

_____

Effect: _____

_____

Graphic notes on anatomical reference model

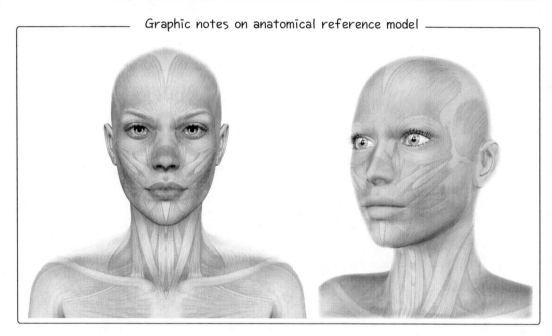

Photo

Graphic notes

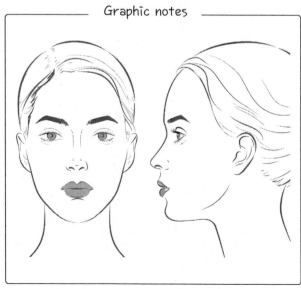

Tape: Quantity _____ Length _____ Width _____ N°Fingers _____ Width. Fingers _____

───────────── Draw the tape ─────────────

How to apply it: _____

_____

_____

_____

_____

_____

_____

_____

_____

_____

_____

_____

_____

_____

Notes: _____

_____

_____

_____

Mark the muscles involved

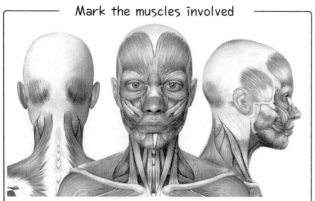

Muscles involved: _____
_____
_____

Application for: _____
_____
_____

Effect: _____
_____

Graphic notes on anatomical reference model

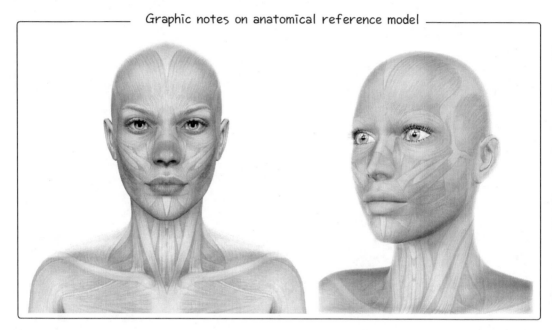

Photo

Graphic notes

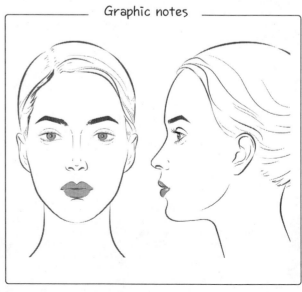

Tape: Quantity _____ Length _____ Width _____ N°Fingers _____ Width. Fingers _____

──────────── Draw the tape ────────────

How to apply it: _____

_____

_____

_____

_____

_____

_____

_____

_____

_____

_____

_____

_____

_____

Notes: _____

_____

_____

_____

Mark the muscles involved

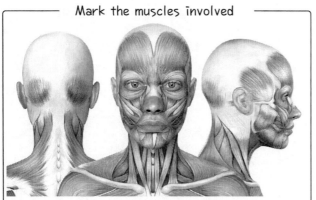

Muscles involved: _____
_____
_____

Application for: _____
_____
_____
_____

Effect: _____
_____

Graphic notes on anatomical reference model

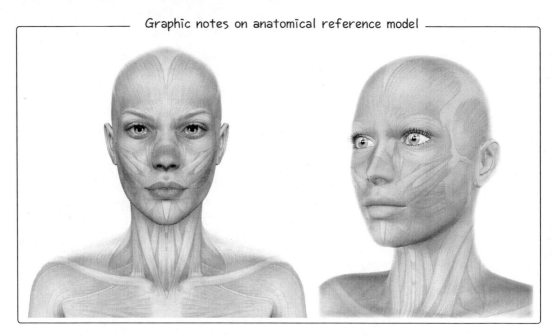

Photo

Graphic notes

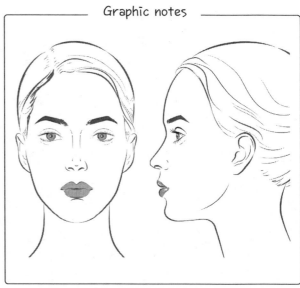

Tape: Quantity _____ Length _____ Width _____ N°Fingers _____ Width. Fingers _____

─────────────── Draw the tape ───────────────

How to apply it: _____

_____

_____

_____

_____

_____

_____

_____

_____

_____

_____

_____

_____

Notes: _____

_____

_____

_____

Mark the muscles involved

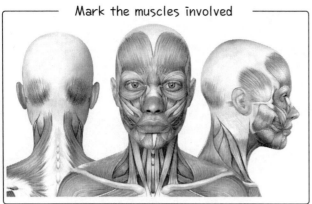

Muscles involved: _____
_____
_____

Application for: _____
_____
_____
_____

Effect:_____
_____

Graphic notes on anatomical reference model

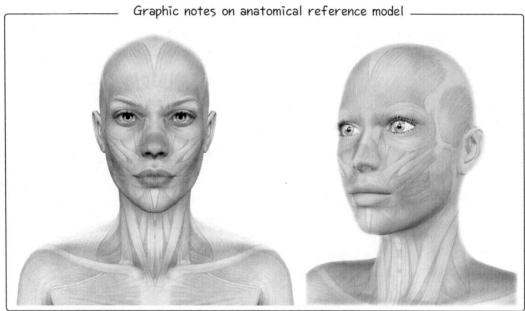

Photo

Graphic notes

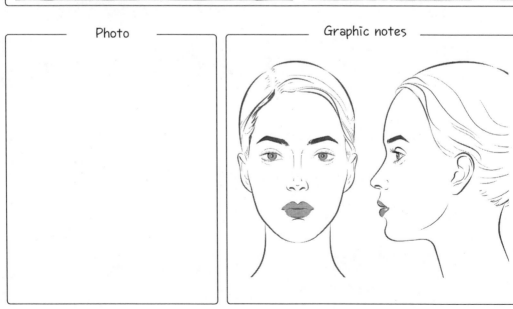

Tape: Quantity _____ Length _____ Width _____ N°Fingers _____ Width. Fingers _____

──────────────── Draw the tape ────────────────

How to apply it: _____

_____

_____

_____

_____

_____

_____

_____

_____

_____

_____

_____

_____

_____

Notes: _____

_____

_____

_____

Mark the muscles involved

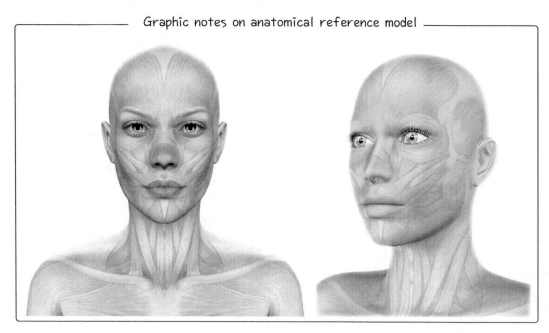

Muscles involved: _____
_____
_____

Application for: _____
_____
_____
_____

Effect: _____
_____
_____

Graphic notes on anatomical reference model

Photo

Graphic notes

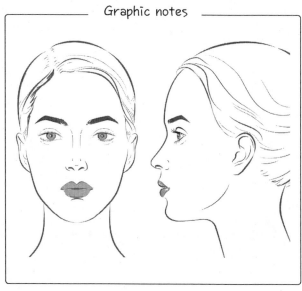

Tape: Quantity _____ Length _____ Width _____ N°Fingers _____ Width. Fingers _____

───────────── Draw the tape ─────────────

How to apply it: _____

_____

_____

_____

_____

_____

_____

_____

_____

_____

_____

_____

Notes: _____

_____

_____

_____

Mark the muscles involved

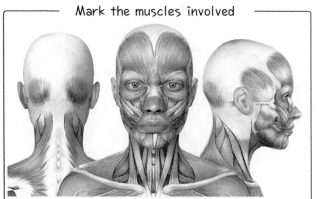

Muscles involved: _____
_____
_____

Application for: _____
_____
_____
_____

Effect: _____
_____

Graphic notes on anatomical reference model

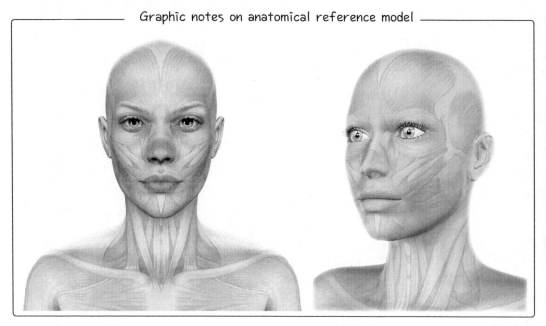

Photo

Graphic notes

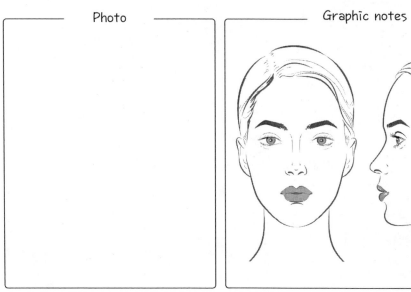

Tape: Quantity _____ Length _____ Width _____ N°Fingers _____ Width. Fingers _____

―――――――――――― Draw the tape ――――――

How to apply it: _____

_____

_____

_____

_____

_____

_____

_____

_____

_____

_____

_____

_____

_____

_____

Notes: _____

_____

_____

_____

Mark the muscles involved

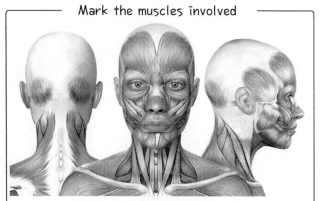

Muscles involved: _____

_____

_____

Application for: _____

_____

_____

Effect: _____

_____

Graphic notes on anatomical reference model

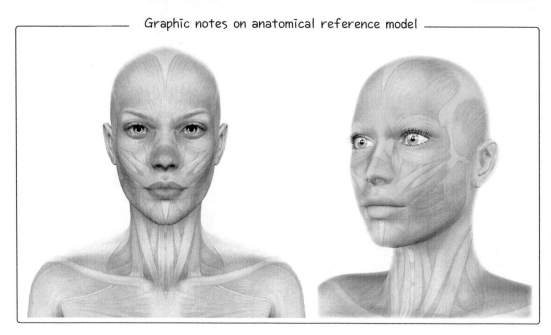

Photo

Graphic notes

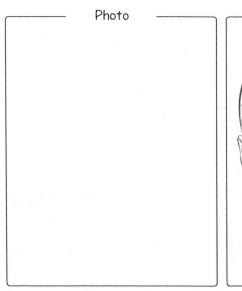

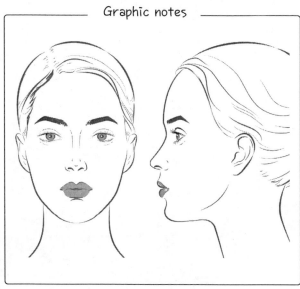

Tape: Quantity _____ Length _____ Width _____ N°Fingers _____ Width. Fingers _____

────── Draw the tape ──────

How to apply it: _____

_____

_____

_____

_____

_____

_____

_____

_____

_____

_____

_____

_____

Notes: _____

_____

_____

_____

Mark the muscles involved

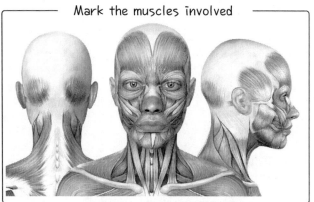

Muscles involved: _____
_____
_____

Application for: _____
_____
_____
_____

Effect: _____
_____

Graphic notes on anatomical reference model

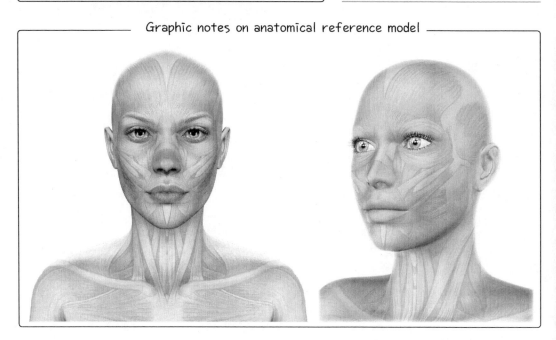

Photo

Graphic notes

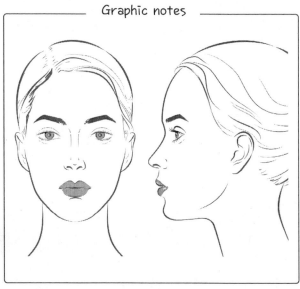

Tape: Quantity _____ Length _____ Width _____ N°Fingers _____ Width. Fingers _____

───── Draw the tape ─────

How to apply it: _____

_____

_____

_____

_____

_____

_____

_____

_____

_____

_____

_____

_____

_____

_____

Notes: _____

_____

_____

_____

Mark the muscles involved

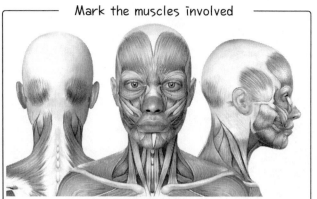

Muscles involved: _____

_____

_____

Application for: _____

_____

_____

_____

Effect: _____

_____

Graphic notes on anatomical reference model

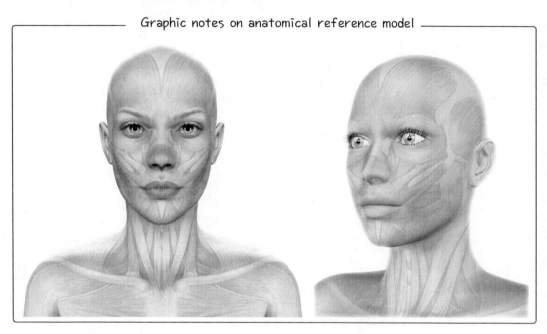

Photo

Graphic notes

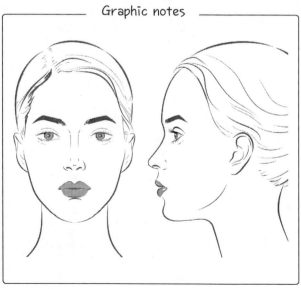

Tape: Quantity _____ Length _____ Width _____ N°Fingers _____ Width. Fingers _____

— Draw the tape —

How to apply it: _____

_____

_____

_____

_____

_____

_____

_____

_____

_____

_____

_____

_____

_____

_____

Notes: _____

_____

_____

_____

Mark the muscles involved

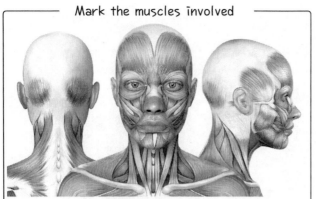

Muscles involved: _____

_____

_____

Application for: _____

_____

_____

Effect:_____

_____

Graphic notes on anatomical reference model

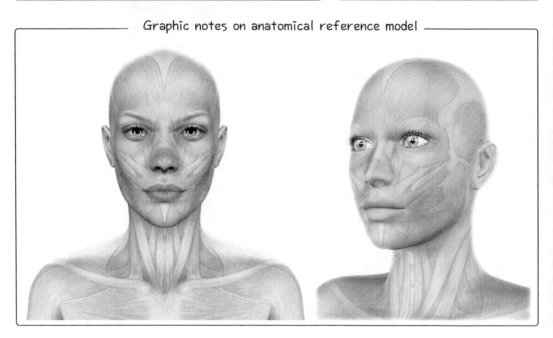

Photo

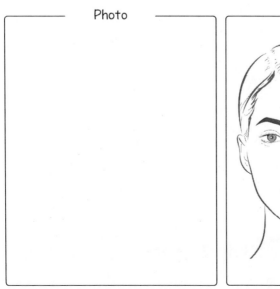

Graphic notes

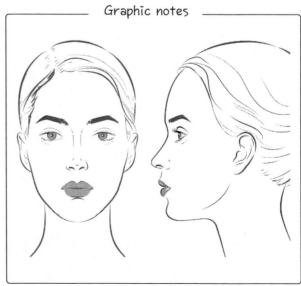

Tape: Quantity _____ Length _____ Width _____ N°Fingers _____ Width. Fingers _____

─── Draw the tape ───

How to apply it: _____

_____

_____

_____

_____

_____

_____

_____

_____

_____

_____

_____

_____

_____

_____

Notes: _____

_____

_____

_____

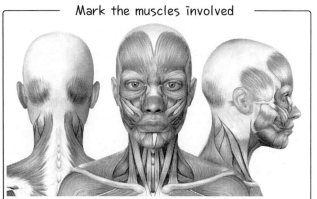

Mark the muscles involved

Muscles involved: _____
_____
_____

Application for: _____
_____
_____
_____

Effect: _____
_____

Graphic notes on anatomical reference model

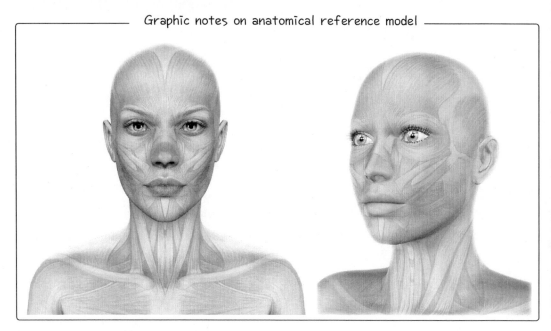

Photo

Graphic notes

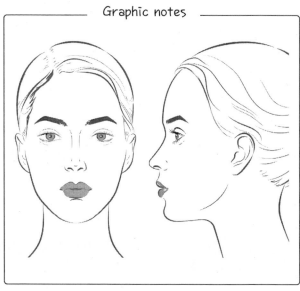

Tape: Quantity _____ Length _____ Width _____ N°Fingers _____ Width. Fingers _____

---------------------------------- Draw the tape ----------------------------------

How to apply it: _____

_____

_____

_____

_____

_____

_____

_____

_____

_____

_____

_____

_____

_____

_____

Notes: _____

_____

_____

_____

Mark the muscles involved

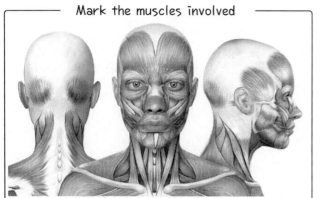

Muscles involved: _____
_____
_____

Application for: _____
_____
_____

Effect: _____
_____

Graphic notes on anatomical reference model

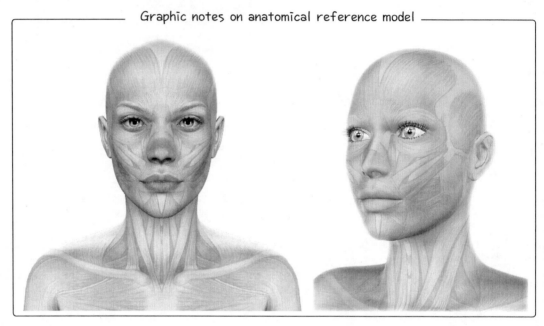

Photo

Graphic notes

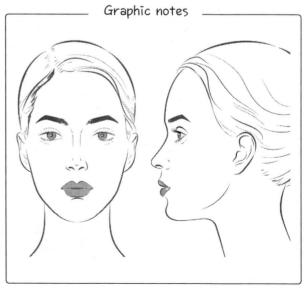

Tape: Quantity _____ Length _____ Width _____ N°Fingers _____ Width. Fingers _____

───────────────── Draw the tape ─────────────────

How to apply it: _____

_____

_____

_____

_____

_____

_____

_____

_____

_____

_____

_____

_____

_____

Notes: _____

_____

_____

_____

Mark the muscles involved

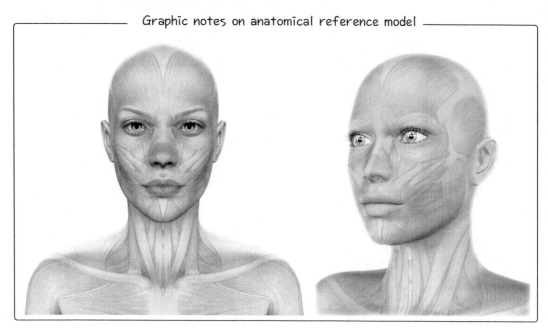

Muscles involved: _____

_____

_____

Application for: _____

_____

_____

_____

Effect: _____

_____

Graphic notes on anatomical reference model

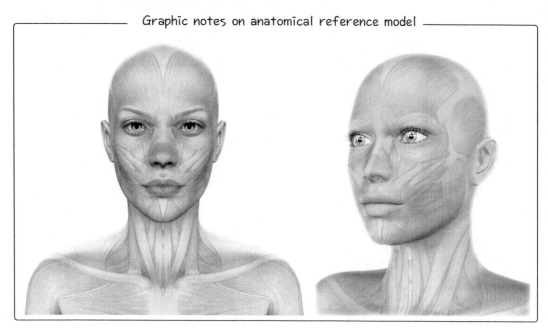

Photo

Graphic notes

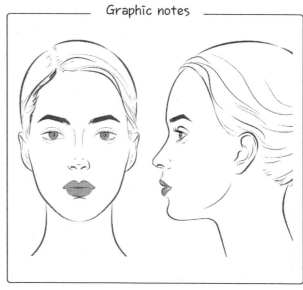

Tape: Quantity _____ Length _____ Width _____ N°Fingers _____ Width. Fingers _____

―――――――――― Draw the tape ――――――――――

How to apply it: _____

_____

_____

_____

_____

_____

_____

_____

_____

_____

_____

_____

_____

_____

Notes: _____

_____

_____

_____

Mark the muscles involved

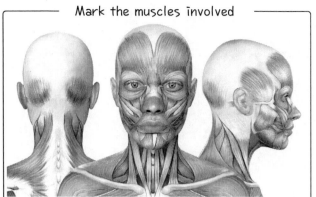

Muscles involved: _____

_____

_____

Application for: _____

_____

_____

Effect: _____

_____

Graphic notes on anatomical reference model

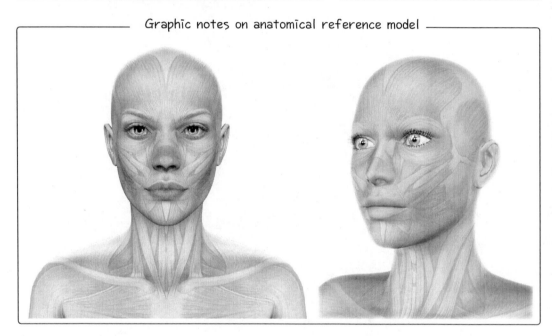

Photo

Graphic notes

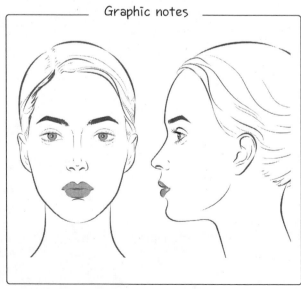

Tape: Quantity _____ Length _____ Width _____ N°Fingers _____ Width. Fingers _____

─── Draw the tape ───

How to apply it: _____

_____

_____

_____

_____

_____

_____

_____

_____

_____

_____

_____

_____

_____

_____

Notes: _____

_____

_____

_____

Mark the muscles involved

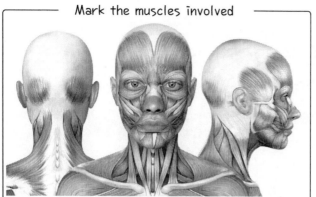

Muscles involved: _____
_____
_____

Application for: _____
_____
_____
_____

Effect: _____
_____

Graphic notes on anatomical reference model

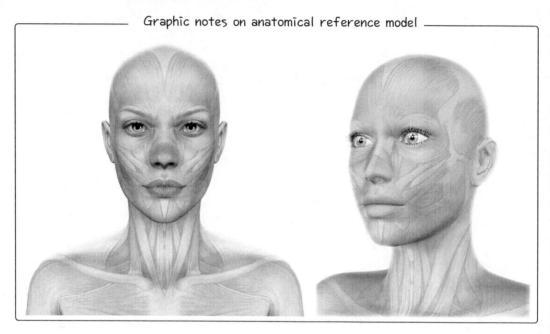

Photo

Graphic notes

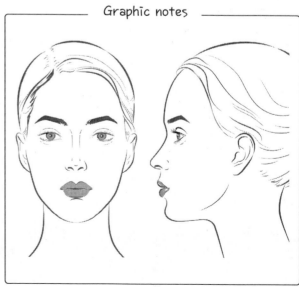

Tape: Quantity _____ Length _____ Width _____ N°Fingers _____ Width. Fingers _____

─────── Draw the tape ───────

How to apply it: _____

_____

_____

_____

_____

_____

_____

_____

_____

_____

_____

_____

_____

_____

Notes: _____

_____

_____

_____

Mark the muscles involved

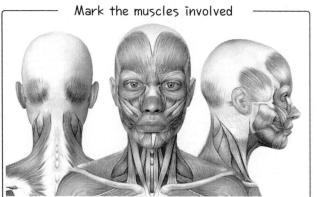

Muscles involved: _____

_____

_____

Application for: _____

_____

_____

_____

Effect:_____

_____

Graphic notes on anatomical reference model

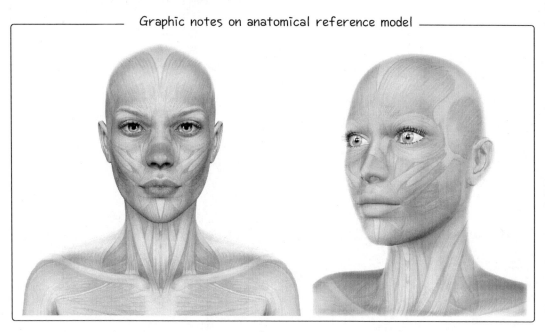

Photo

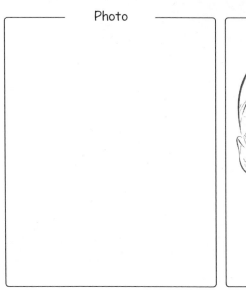

Graphic notes

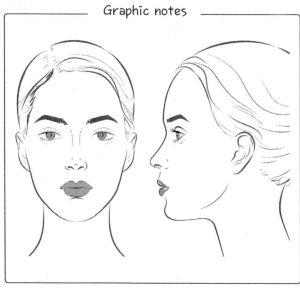

Tape: Quantity _____ Length _____ Width _____ N°Fingers _____ Width. Fingers _____

─────────────── Draw the tape ───────────────

How to apply it: _____

_____

_____

_____

_____

_____

_____

_____

_____

_____

_____

_____

_____

_____

Notes: _____

_____

_____

_____

Mark the muscles involved

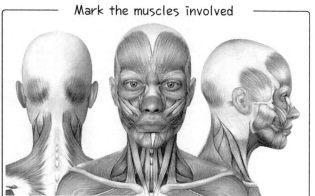

Muscles involved: _____
_____
_____

Application for: _____
_____
_____
_____

Effect: _____
_____

Graphic notes on anatomical reference model

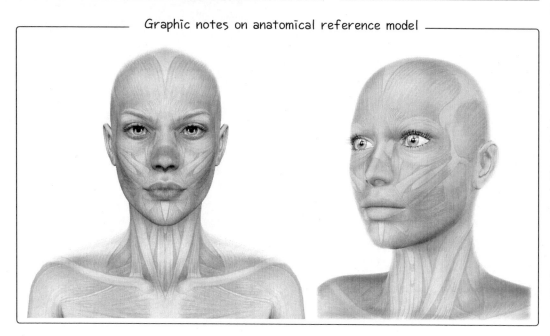

Photo

Graphic notes

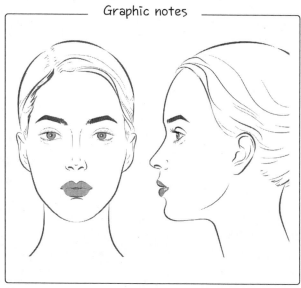

Tape: Quantity _____ Length _____ Width _____ N°Fingers _____ Width. Fingers _____

---------- Draw the tape ----------

How to apply it: _____

_____

_____

_____

_____

_____

_____

_____

_____

_____

_____

_____

_____

_____

Notes: _____

_____

_____

_____

Mark the muscles involved

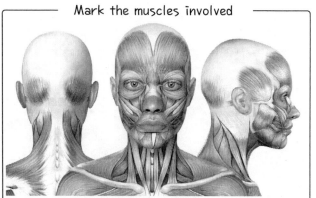

Muscles involved: _____
_____
_____

Application for: _____
_____
_____

Effect: _____
_____

Graphic notes on anatomical reference model

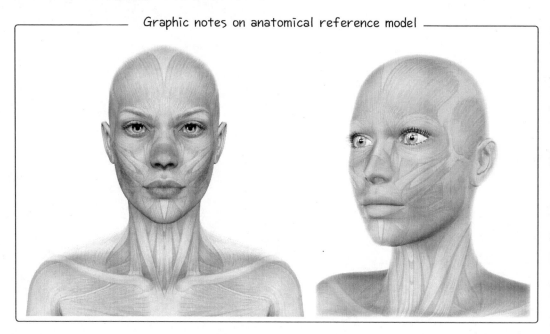

Photo

Graphic notes

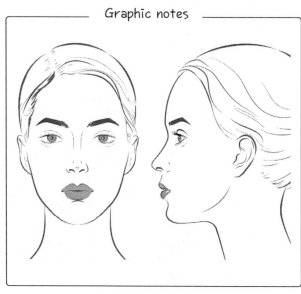

Tape: Quantity _____ Length _____ Width _____ N°Fingers _____ Width. Fingers _____

──────────── Draw the tape ────────────

How to apply it: _____

_____

_____

_____

_____

_____

_____

_____

_____

_____

_____

_____

_____

_____

_____

Notes: _____

_____

_____

_____

Mark the muscles involved

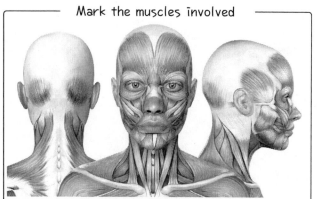

Muscles involved: _____
_____
_____

Application for: _____
_____
_____
_____

Effect: _____
_____

Graphic notes on anatomical reference model

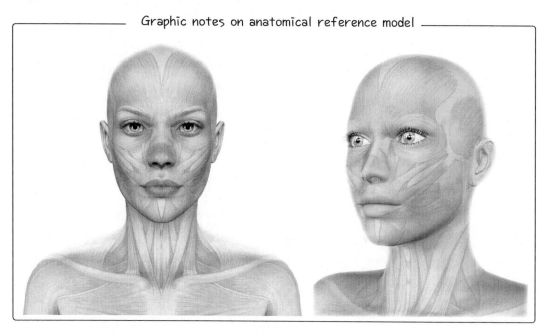

Photo

Graphic notes

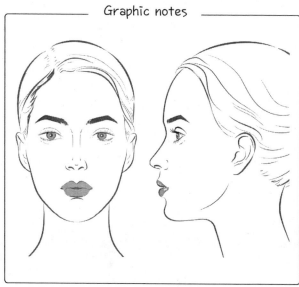

Tape: Quantity _____ Length _____ Width _____ N°Fingers _____ Width. Fingers _____

─────────────── Draw the tape ───────────────

How to apply it: _____

_____

_____

_____

_____

_____

_____

_____

_____

_____

_____

_____

_____

Notes: _____

_____

_____

_____

Mark the muscles involved

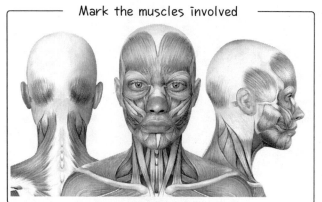

Muscles involved: _____

_____

_____

Application for: _____

_____

_____

_____

Effect: _____

_____

Graphic notes on anatomical reference model

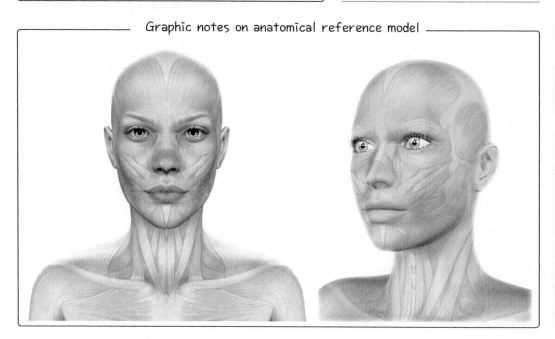

Photo

Graphic notes

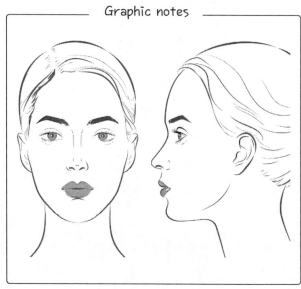

Tape: Quantity _____ Length _____ Width _____ N°Fingers _____ Width. Fingers _____

Draw the tape

How to apply it: _____

_____

_____

_____

_____

_____

_____

_____

_____

_____

_____

_____

_____

_____

_____

_____

Notes: _____

_____

_____

_____

Me before

Me after

Made in United States
North Haven, CT
05 December 2024

61800665R00054